Keto Chaffle Recipes Cookbook 2022:

The last cookbook with the most wanted and updated recipes to lose weight fast and regain confidence in a few steps

SARAH BUCKLEY

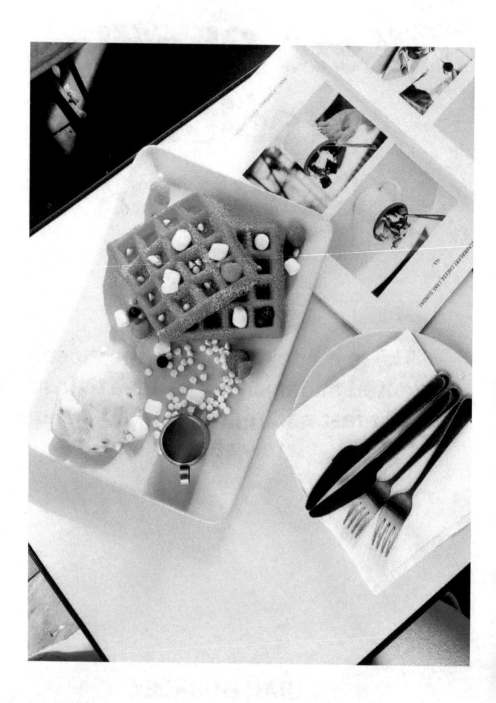

Legal & Disclaimer

The information contained in this book and its contents is not designed to replace or take the place of any form of medical or professional advice; and is not meant to replace the need for independent medical, financial, legal or other professional advice or services, as may be required. The content and information in this book have been provided for educational and entertainment purposes only.

The content and information contained in this book have been compiled from sources deemed reliable, and it is accurate to the best of the Author's knowledge, information, and belief. However, the author cannot guarantee its accuracy and validity and cannot be held liable for any errors and/or omissions. Further, changes are periodically made to this book as and when needed. Where appropriate and/or necessary, you must consult a professional (including but not limited to your doctor, attorney, financial advisor or such other professional advisor) before using any of the suggested remedies, techniques, or information in this book.

Upon using the contents and information contained in this book, you agree to hold harmless the Author from and against any damages, costs, and expenses, including any legal fees potentially resulting from the application of any of the information provided by this

TABLE OF CONTENTS

INTRODUCTION

Whether you want to lose some weight or burn fat, you can use keto chaff in your diet plan. Keto chaff is a dietary supplement that contains no calories or carbohydrates. It contains low carbohydrates and also low calories. A keto flail is supposed to help with weight loss.

How it works: The chaffle is made of shredded coconut and pumpkin seeds. It works by providing a low-calorie carbohydrate source that fuels your body while keeping your blood sugar stable. When you continue to use the chaff, it helps to suppress hunger and increase fat burning.

Chaffle is made with coconut and pumpkin, making it a healthy low-carb alternative for anyone looking to lose weight. As part of a healthy diet, the chaffle helps stabilise blood sugar levels, making it easier for the body to recognise when it needs nourishment. Keto Chaffle contains no calories or carbohydrates, making it an ideal tool for anyone looking to lose or maintain weight.

Regularly, keto dieters keep an eye out for ways to stick to the diet exactly, while also looking for ways to make life easier.

Chaffles are one of those foods that have a stimulating effect on the low-carb lifestyle. I find them to be an easy solution, and fortunately they can be enjoyed at different times of the day. In the recipes below, I show many ways you can prepare and use Chaffles - for breakfast to dinner, as a snack and as a dessert.

So, this mix makes dieting easier because chaffles are loaded with healthy fats and mostly contain no carbs. Achieving ketosis just got easier!

Lastly, they are convenient for meal prepping ahead of time. And we know how meal prepping helps with an effective keto diet. Chaffles can be frozen for later use, and they taste great when reheated and enjoyed later.

Once you get hooked on Chaffles, they will become an important part of your diet because of the benefits they bring. I've been making them non-stop for weeks now, and am thinking of creating a second cookbook with my new chaffle discoveries.

How to Make Chaffles?

Equipment and Ingredients Discussed

Making chaffles requires five simple steps and nothing more than a waffle maker for flat chaffles and a waffle bowl maker for chaffle bowls.

To make chaffles, you will need two necessary ingredients – eggs and cheese. My preferred cheeses are cheddar cheese or mozzarella cheese. These melt quickly, making them the go-to for most recipes. Meanwhile, always ensure that your cheeses are finely grated or thinly sliced for use.

Now, to make a standard chaffle:

- First, preheat your waffle maker until adequately hot.

- Meanwhile, in a bowl, mix the egg with cheese on hand until well combined.

- Open the iron, pour in a quarter or half of the mixture, and close.

- Cook the chaffle for 5 to 7 minutes or until it is crispy.

- Transfer the chaffle to a plate and allow cooling before serving.

11 Tips to Make Chaffles

My surefire ways to turn out the crispiest of chaffles:

- **Preheat Well:** Yes! It sounds obvious to preheat the waffle iron before usage. However, preheating the iron moderately will not get your chaffles as crispy as you will like. The best way to preheat before cooking is to ensure that the iron is very hot.

- **Not-So-Cheesy:** Will you prefer to have your chaffles less cheesy? Then, use mozzarella cheese.

- **Not-So Eggy**: If you aren't comfortable with the smell of eggs in your chaffles, try using egg whites instead of egg yolks or whole eggs.

- **To Shred or to Slice:** Many recipes call for shredded cheese when making chaffles, but I find sliced cheeses to offer crispier pieces. While I stick with mostly shredded cheese for convenience's sake, be at ease to use sliced cheese in the same quantity. When using sliced cheeses, arrange two to four pieces in the waffle iron, top with the beaten eggs, and some slices of the cheese. Cover and cook until crispy.

- **Shallower Irons:** For better crisps on your chaffles, use shallower waffle irons as they cook easier and faster.

- **Layering:** Don't fill up the waffle iron with too much batter. Work between a quarter and a half cup of total ingredients per batch for correctly done chaffles.

- **Patience:** It is a virtue even when making chaffles. For the best results, allow the chaffles to sit in the iron for 5 to 7 minutes before serving.

- **No Peeking:** 7 minutes isn't too much of a time to wait for the outcome of your chaffles, in my opinion. Opening the iron and checking on the chaffle before it is done stands you a worse chance of ruining it.

- **Crispy Cooling:** For better crisp, I find that allowing the chaffles to cool further after they are transferred to a plate aids a lot.

- **Easy Cleaning:** For the best cleanup, wet a paper towel and wipe the inner parts of the iron clean while still warm. Kindly note that the iron should be warm but not hot!

- **Brush It:** Also, use a clean toothbrush to clean between the iron's teeth for a thorough cleanup. You may also use a dry, rough sponge to clean the iron while it is still warm

SPECIAL CHAFFLE RECIPES

1. Breakfast Spinach Ricotta Chaffles

Preparation time: 8 minutes

Cooking Time: 28 Minutes

Servings: 2

Ingredients:

- 4 oz frozen spinach, thawed, squeezed dry
- 1 cup ricotta cheese
- 2 eggs, beaten
- ½ tsp garlic powder
- ¼ cup finely grated Pecorino Romano cheese
- ½ cup finely grated mozzarella cheese
- Salt and freshly ground black pepper to taste

Directions:

1. Preheat the waffle iron.
2. In a medium bowl, mix all the ingredients.
3. Open the iron, lightly grease with cooking spray and spoon in a quarter of the mixture.
4. Close the iron and cook until brown and crispy, 7 minutes.

5. Remove the chaffle onto a plate and set aside.

6. Make three more chaffles with the remaining mixture.

7. Allow cooling and serve afterward.

Nutrition: Calories 1Fats 13.15gCarbs 5.06gNet Carbs 4.06gProtein 12.79g

2. Pumpkin Chaffle With Frosting

Preparation time: 10 minutes

Cooking Time: 15 Minutes

Servings: 2

Ingredients:

- 1 egg, lightly beaten
- 1 tbsp sugar-free pumpkin puree
- 1/4 tsp pumpkin pie spice
- 1/2 cup mozzarella cheese, shredded
- For frosting:
- 1/2 tsp vanilla
- 2 tbsp Swerve
- 2 tbsp cream cheese, softened

Directions:

1. Preheat your waffle maker.
2. Add egg in a bowl and whisk well.
3. Add pumpkin puree, pumpkin pie spice, and cheese and stir well.
4. Spray waffle maker with cooking spray.

5. Pour 1/2 of the batter in the hot waffle maker and cook for 3-4 minutes or until golden brown. Repeat with the remaining batter.
6. In a small bowl, mix all frosting ingredients until smooth.
7. Add frosting on top of hot chaffles and serve.

Nutrition: Calories 9at 7 carbohydrates 3.6 sugar 0.6 protein 5.6 cholesterol 97 mg

3. Chaffle Strawbery Sandwich

Preparation time: 7 minutes

Cooking Time: 5 Minutes

Servings: 2

Ingredients:

- 1/4 cup heavy cream
- 4 oz. strawberry slice
- CHAFFLE Ingredients:
- 1 egg
- ½ cup mozzarella cheese

Directions:

1. Make 2 chaffles with chaffle ingredients
2. Meanwhile, mix together cream and strawberries.
3. Spread this mixture over chaffle slice.
4. Drizzle chocolate sauce over a sandwich.
5. Serve and enjoy!

Nutrition: Protein: 18% 4kcal Fat: 78% 196 kcal Carbohydrates: 4% 10 kcal

4. Chocolate Chaffle

Preparation time: 10 minutes

Cooking Time: 8 Minutes

Ingredients:

- 1 egg
- ½ cup mozzarella cheese, shredded
- ½ teaspoon baking powder
- 2 tablespoons cocoa powder
- 2 tablespoons sweetener
- 2 tablespoons almond flour

Directions:

1. Turn your waffle maker on.
2. Beat the egg in a bowl.
3. Stir in the rest of the ingredients.
4. Put the mixture into the waffle maker.
5. Seal the device and cook for 4 minutes.
6. Open and transfer the chaffle to a plate to cool for 2 minutes.
7. Do the same steps using the remaining mixture.

Nutrition: Calories 149 Total Fat 10. Saturated Fat 2.4g Cholesterol 86mg Sodium 80mg Potassium

291mg Total Carbohydrate 9g Dietary Fiber 4.1g Protein 8.8g Total Sugars 0.3g

5. New Year Keto Chaffle Cake

Servings:5

Cooking Time:15minutes

Ingredients:

- 4 oz. almond flour
- 2 cup cheddar cheese
- 5 eggs
- 1 tsp. stevia
- 2 tsp baking powder
- 2 tsp vanilla extract
- 1/4 cup almond butter, melted
- 3 tbsps. almond milk
- 1 cup cranberries
- I cup coconut cream

Directions:

1. Crack eggs in a small mixing bowl, mix the eggs, almond flour, stevia, and baking powder.
2. Add the melted butter slowly to the flour mixture, mix well to ensure a smooth consistency.
3. Add the cheese, almond milk, cranberries and vanilla to the flour and butter mixture be sure to mix well.

4. Preheat waffles maker according to manufacturer instruction and grease it with avocado oil.
5. Pour mixture into waffle maker and cook until golden brown.
6. Make 5 chaffles
7. Stag chaffles in a plate. Spread the cream all around.
8. Cut in slice and serve.

Nutrition: Protein: 3% 15 Kcal Fat: % 207 Kcal Carbohydrates: 3% 15 Kcal

6. Thanksgiving Pumpkin Latte with Chaffles

Preparation time: 10 minutes

Cooking Time:5minutes

Servings: 2

Ingredients:

- 3/4 cup unsweetened coconut milk
- 2 tbsps. Heavy cream
- 2 tbsps. Pumpkin puree
- 1 tsp. stevia
- 1/4 tsp pumpkin spice
- 1/4 tsp Vanilla extract
- 1/4 cup espresso
- FOR TOPPING
- 2 scoop whipped cream
- Pumpkin spice
- 2 heart shape minutes chaffles

Directions:

1. Mix together all recipe ingredients in mug and microwave for minutes Ute.
2. Pour the latte into a serving glass.

3. Top with a heavy cream scoop, pumpkin spice, and chaffle.

4. Serve and enjoy!

Nutrition: Protein: 16 kcal Fat: 85% 259 kcal Carbohydrates: 10% 29 kcal

7. Choco And Strawberries Chaffles

Preparation time: 10 minutes

Cooking Time:5 minutes

Servings: 2

Ingredients:

- 1 tbsp. almond flour
- 1/2 cup strawberry puree
- 1/2 cup cheddar cheese
- 1 tbsp. cocoa powder
- ½ tsp baking powder
- 1 large egg.
- 2 tbsps. coconut oil. melted
- 1/2 tsp vanilla extract optional

Directions:

1. Preheat waffle iron while you are mixing the ingredients.
2. Melt oil in a microwave.
3. In a small mixing bowl, mix together flour, baking powder, flour, and vanilla until well combined.
4. Add egg, melted oil, ½ cup cheese and strawberry puree to the flour mixture.

5. Pour 1/8 cup cheese in a waffle maker and then pour the mixture in the center of greased waffle.

6. Again, sprinkle cheese on the batter.

7. Close the waffle maker.

8. Cook chaffles for about 4-5 minutes Utes until cooked and crispy.

9. Once chaffles are cooked, remove and enjoy!

Nutrition: Protein: 15% 48 kcal Fat: 79% 246 kcal Carbohydrates: 5% 17 kcal

8. Lemon and Paprika Chaffles

Preparation time: 8 minutes

Cooking Time: 28 Minutes

Servings: 2

Ingredients:

- 1 egg, beaten
- 1 oz cream cheese, softened
- 1/3 cup finely grated mozzarella cheese
- 1 tbsp almond flour
- 1 tsp butter, melted
- 1 tsp maple (sugar-free) syrup
- ½ tsp sweet paprika
- ½ tsp lemon extract

Directions:

1. Preheat the waffle iron.
2. Mix all the ingredients in a medium bowl
3. Open the iron and pour in a quarter of the mixture. Close and cook until crispy, 7 minutes.
4. Remove the chaffle onto a plate and make 3 more with the remaining mixture.

5. Cut each chaffle into wedges, plate, allow cooling and serve.

Nutrition: Calories 48Fats 4.22gCarbs 0.Net Carbs 0.5gProtein 2g

9. Triple Chocolate Chaffle

Preparation time: 5 minutes

Cooking Time:7–9 Minutes

Servings: 2

Ingredients:

- Batter
- 4 eggs
- 4 ounces cream cheese, softened
- 1 ounce dark unsweetened chocolate, melted
- 1 teaspoon vanilla extract
- 5 tablespoons almond flour
- 3 tablespoons cocoa powder
- 1½ teaspoons baking powder
- ¼ cup dark unsweetened chocolate chips
- Other
- 2 tablespoons butter to brush the waffle maker

Directions:

1. Preheat the waffle maker.
2. Add the eggs and cream cheese to a bowl and stir with a wire whisk until just combined.
3. Add the vanilla extract and mix until combined.

4. Stir in the almond flour, cocoa powder, and baking powder and mix until combined.

5. Add the chocolate chips and stir.

6. Brush the heated waffle maker with butter and add a few tablespoons of the batter.

7. Close the lid and cook for about 8 minutes depending on your waffle maker.

8. Serve and enjoy.

Nutrition: Calories 385, fat 33 g, carbs 10.6 g, sugar 0.7 g, Protein 12.g, sodium 199 mg

10. <u>Basic Chaffle</u>

Preparation time: 10 minutes

Cooking Time: 8 Minutes

Servings: 2

Ingredients:

- Cooking spray
- 1 egg
- ½ cup cheddar cheese, shredded

Directions:

1. Turn your waffle maker on.
2. Grease both sides with cooking spray.
3. Beat the egg in a bowl.
4. Stir in the cheddar cheese.
5. Pour half of the batter into the waffle maker.
6. Seal and cook for 4 minutes.
7. Remove the chaffle slowly from the waffle maker.
8. Let sit for 3 minutes.
9. Pour the remaining batter into the waffle maker and repeat the steps.

Nutrition: Calories 191 Total Fat 23 g Saturated Fat 14 g Cholesterol 223 mg Sodium 413 mg Potassium 116 mg   Total Carbohydrate 1 g   Dietary Fiber 1 g   Protein 20 g Total Sugars 1 g

11. **Nut Butter Chaffle**

Preparation time: 10 minutes

Cooking Time: 8 Minutes

Servings: 2

Ingredients:

- 1 egg
- ½ cup mozzarella cheese, shredded
- 2 tablespoons almond flour
- ½ teaspoon baking powder
- 1 tablespoon sweetener
- 1 teaspoon vanilla
- 2 tablespoons nut butter

Directions:

1. Turn on the waffle maker.
2. Beat the egg in a bowl and combine with the cheese.
3. In another bowl, mix the almond flour, baking powder and sweetener.
4. In the third bowl, blend the vanilla extract and nut butter.
5. Gradually add the almond flour mixture into the egg mixture.

6. Then, stir in the vanilla extract.

7. Pour the batter into the waffle maker.

8. Cook for 4 minutes.

9. Transfer to a plate and let cool for 2 minutes.

10. Repeat the steps with the remaining batter.

Nutrition: Calories 168 Total Fat 15.5g Saturated Fat 3.9g Cholesterol 34mg Sodium 31mg Potassium 64mg Total Carbohydrate 1.6gDietary Fiber 1.4g Protein 5.4g Total Sugars 0.6g

12. **Keto Coffee Chaffles**

Preparation time: 10 minutes

Cooking Time:5 minutes

Servings: 2

Ingredients:

- 1 tbsp. almond flour
- 1 tbsp. instant coffee
- 1/2 cup cheddar cheese
- ½ tsp baking powder
- 1 large egg

Directions:

1. Preheat waffle iron and grease with cooking spray
2. Meanwhile, in a small mixing bowl, mix together all ingredients and ½ cup cheese.
3. Pour 1/8 cup cheese in a waffle maker and then pour the mixture in the center of greased waffle.
4. Again, sprinkle cheese on the batter.
5. Close the waffle maker.
6. Cook chaffles for about 4-5 minutes Utes until cooked and crispy.
7. Once chaffles are cooked, remove and enjoy!

Nutrition: Protein: 26% 47 kcal Fat: 69% 125 kcal Carbohydrates: 5% 9 kcal

13. Chaffle Ice Cream Bowl

Preparation time: 10 minutes

Cooking Time: 0 Minutes

Servings: 2

Ingredients:

- 4 basic chaffles
- 2 scoops keto ice cream
- 2 teaspoons sugar-free chocolate syrup

Directions:

1. Arrange 2 basic chaffles in a bowl, following the contoured design of the bowl.
2. Top with the ice cream.
3. Drizzle with the syrup on top.
4. Serve.

Nutrition: Calories 181 Total Fat 17.2g Saturated Fat 4.2g Cholesterol 26mg Sodium 38mg Total Carbohydrate 7g Dietary Fiber 1g Total Sugars 4.1g Protein 0.4g Potassium 0mg

14. Peanut Butter Sandwich Chaffle

Preparation time: 10 minutes

Cooking Time: 15 Minutes

Servings: 2

Ingredients:

- For chaffle:
- 1 egg, lightly beaten
- 1/2 cup mozzarella cheese, shredded
- 1/4 tsp espresso powder
- 1 tbsp unsweetened chocolate chips
- 1 tbsp Swerve
- 2 tbsp unsweetened cocoa powder
- For filling:
- 1 tbsp butter, softened
- 2 tbsp Swerve
- 3 tbsp creamy peanut butter

Directions:

1. Preheat your waffle maker.
2. In a bowl, whisk together egg, espresso powder, chocolate chips, Swerve, and cocoa powder.
3. Add mozzarella cheese and stir well.

4. Spray waffle maker with cooking spray.

5. Pour 1/2 of the batter in the hot waffle maker and cook for 3-4 minutes or until golden brown. Repeat with the remaining batter.

6. For filling: In a small bowl, stir together butter, Swerve, and peanut butter until smooth.

7. Once chaffles is cool, then spread filling mixture between two chaffle and place in the fridge for 10 minutes.

8. Cut chaffle sandwich in half and serve.

Nutrition: Calories 1Fat 16.1 carbohydrates 9.6 sugar 1.1 protein 8.2 cholesterol 101 mg

15. <u>Chocolate Chaffle Rolls</u>

Preparation time: 7 minutes

Cooking Time: 10 Minutes

Servings: 2

Ingredients:

- 1/2 cup mozzarella cheese
- 1 tbsp. almond flour
- 1 egg
- 1 tsp cinnamon
- 1 tsp stevia
- FILLING
- 1 tbsp. coconut cream
- 1 tbsp. coconut flour
- 1/4 cup keto chocolate chips

Directions:

1. Switch on a round waffle maker and let it heat up.
2. In a small bowl, mix together cheese, egg, flour, cinnamon powder, and stevia in a bowl.
3. Spray the round waffle maker with nonstick spray.
4. Pour the batter in a waffle maker and close the lid.

5. Close the waffle maker and cook for about 3-4 minutes Utes.

6. Once chaffles are cooked remove from Maker

7. Meanwhile, mix together cream flour and chocolate chips in bowl and microwave for 30 sec.

8. Spread this filling over chaffle and roll it.

9. Serve and enjoy!

Nutrition: Protein: 32% 50 kcal Fat: 61% 94 kcal Carbohydrates: 7% 11 kcal

16. Chaffles Ice-cream Topping

Preparation time: 7 minutes

Cooking Time: 5 Minutes

Servings: 2

Ingredients:

- 1/4 cup coconut cream, frozen
- 1 cup coconut flour
- ¼ cup strawberries chunks
- 1 tsp. vanilla extract
- 1 oz. chocolate flakes
- 4 keto chaffles

Directions:

1. Mix together all ingredients in a mixing bowl.
2. Spread mixture between chaffles and freeze in the freezer for 2 hours.
3. Serve chill and enjoy!

Nutrition: Protein: 26% 68 kcal Fat: 71% 187 kcal Carbohydrates: 3% 9 kcal

17. **Easter Morning Simple Chaffles**

Preparation time: 7 minutes

Cooking Time:5minutes

Servings: 2

Ingredients:

- 1/2 cup egg whites
- 1 cup mozzarella cheese, melted

Directions:

1. Switch on your square waffle maker. Spray with non-stick spray.
2. Beat egg whites with beater, until fluffy and white.
3. Add cheese and mix well.
4. Pour batter in a waffle maker.
5. Close the maker and cook for about 3 minutes Utes.
6. Repeat with the remaining batter.
7. Remove chaffles from the maker.
8. Serve hot and enjoy!

Nutrition: Protein: 36% 42 kcal Fat: 60% 71 kcal Carbohydrates: 4% 5 kcal

18. Pumpkin Cheesecake Chaffle

Preparation time: 10 minutes

Cooking Time: 15 Minutes

Servings: 2

Ingredients:

- For chaffle:
- 1 egg
- 1/2 tsp vanilla
- 1/2 tsp baking powder, gluten-free
- 1/4 tsp pumpkin spice
- 1 tsp cream cheese, softened
- 2 tsp heavy cream
- 1 tbsp Swerve
- 1 tbsp almond flour
- 2 tsp pumpkin puree
- 1/2 cup mozzarella cheese, shredded
- For filling:
- 1/4 tsp vanilla
- 1 tbsp Swerve
- 2 tbsp cream cheese

Directions:

1. Preheat your mini waffle maker.

2. In a small bowl, mix all chaffle ingredients.

3. Spray waffle maker with cooking spray.

4. Pour half batter in the hot waffle maker and cook for 3-5 minutes. Repeat with the remaining batter.

5. In a small bowl, combine all filling ingredients.

6. Spread filling mixture between two chaffles and place in the fridge for 10 minutes.

7. Serve and enjoy.

Nutrition: Calories 107Fat 7.2 carbohydrates 5 sugar 0.7 protein 6.7 cholesterol 93 mg

19. Cinnamon Chaffle Rolls

Preparation time: 7 minutes

Cooking Time:10 Minutes

Servings: 2

Ingredients:

- 1/2 cup mozzarella cheese
- 1 tbsp. almond flour
- 1 egg
- 1 tsp cinnamon
- 1 tsp stevia
- CINNAMON ROLL GLAZE
- 1 tbsp. butter
- 1 tbsp. cream cheese
- 1 tsp. cinnamon
- 1/4 tsp vanilla extract
- 1 tbsp. coconut flour

Directions:

1. Switch on a round waffle maker and let it heat up.
2. In a small bowl mix together cheese, egg, flour, cinnamon powder, and stevia in a bowl.
3. Spray the round waffle maker with nonstick spray.

4. Pour the batter in a waffle maker and close the lid.

5. Close the waffle maker and cook for about 3-4 minutes Utes.

6. Once chaffles are cooked, remove from Maker

7. Mix together butter, cream cheese, cinnamon, vanilla and coconut flour in a bowl.

8. Spread this glaze over chaffle and roll up.

9. Serve and enjoy!

Nutrition: Protein: 25% 52 kcal Fat: 69% 142 kcal Carbohydrates: 7% 14 kcal

20. Double Chocolate Chaffles

Preparation time: 10 minutes

Cooking Time:5 minutes

Servings: 2

Ingredients:

- 1/4 cup unsweetened chocolate chips
- 2 tbsps. cocoa powder
- 1 cup egg whites
- 1 tsp. coffee powder
- 2 tbsps. almond flour
- 1/2 cup mozzarella cheese
- 1 tbsp. coconut milk
- 1 tsp. baking powder
- 1 tsp. stevia

Directions:

1. Switch on your Belgian chaffle maker.
2. Spray the waffle maker with cooking spray.
3. Beat egg whites with an electric beater until fluffy and white.
4. Add the rest of the ingredients to the egg whites and mix them again.

5. Pour batter in a greased waffle maker and make two fluffy chaffles.

6. Once chaffles are cooked, remove from the maker.

7. Serve with coconut cream, and berries

8. Enjoy!

Nutrition: Protein: 52% kcal Fat: 39% 73 kcal Carbohydrates: 9% 17 kcal

21. **Breakfast Peanut Butter Chaffle**

Preparation time: 10 minutes

Cooking Time: 15 Minutes

Servings: 2

Ingredients:

- 1 egg, lightly beaten
- ½ tsp vanilla
- 1 tbsp Swerve
- 2 tbsp powdered peanut butter
- ½ cup mozzarella cheese, shredded

Directions:

1. Preheat your waffle maker.
2. Add all ingredients into the bowl and mix until well combined.
3. Spray waffle maker with cooking spray.
4. Pour half batter in the hot waffle maker and cook for 5-7 minutes or until golden brown. Repeat with the remaining batter.
5. Serve and enjoy.

Nutrition: Calories 80Fat 4.1 carbohydrates 2.9 sugar 0.gProtein 7.4 cholesterol 86 mg

22. Apple Cinnamon Chaffles

Preparation time: 6 minutes

Cooking Time: 20 Minutes

Servings: 2

Ingredients:

- 3 eggs, lightly beaten
- 1 cup mozzarella cheese, shredded
- ¼ cup apple, chopped
- ½ tsp monk fruit sweetener
- 1 ½ tsp cinnamon
- ¼ tsp baking powder, gluten-free
- 2 tbsp coconut flour

Directions:

1. Preheat your waffle maker.
2. Add remaining ingredients and stir until well combined.
3. Spray waffle maker with cooking spray.
4. Pour 1/3 of batter in the hot waffle maker and cook for minutes or until golden brown. Repeat with the remaining batter.
5. Serve and enjoy.

Nutrition: Calories 142Fat 7.4 carbohydrates 9.7 sugar 3 protein 9.gCholesterol 169 mg

23. <u>Churro Chaffle</u>

Preparation time: 10 minutes

Cooking Time: 8 Minutes

Servings: 2

Ingredients:

- 1 egg
- ½ cup mozzarella cheese, shredded
- ½ teaspoon cinnamon
- 2 tablespoons sweetener

Directions:

1. Turn on your waffle iron.
2. Beat the egg in a bowl.
3. Stir in the cheese.
4. Pour half of the mixture into the waffle maker.
5. Cover the waffle iron.
6. Cook for 4 minutes.
7. While waiting, mix the cinnamon and sweetener in a bowl.
8. Open the device and soak the waffle in the cinnamon mixture.
9. Repeat the steps with the remaining batter.

Nutrition: Calories   Total Fat 6.9g Saturated Fat 2.9g   Cholesterol 171mg   Sodium 147mg   Potassium 64mg Total Carbohydrate 5.8g Dietary Fiber 2.6g Protein 9.6g Total Sugars 0.4g

24. <u>Blueberry Chaffles</u>

Preparation time: 8 minutes

Cooking Time: 15 Minutes

Servings: 2

Ingredients:

- 2 eggs
- 1/2 cup blueberries
- 1/2 tsp baking powder
- 1/2 tsp vanilla
- 2 tsp Swerve
- 3 tbsp almond flour
- 1 cup mozzarella cheese, shredded

Directions:

1. Preheat your waffle maker.
2. In a medium bowl, mix eggs, vanilla, Swerve, almond flour, and cheese.
3. Add blueberries and stir well.
4. Spray waffle maker with cooking spray.
5. Pour 1/4 batter in the hot waffle maker and cook for 8 minutes or until golden brown. Repeat with the remaining batter.

6. Serve and enjoy.

Nutrition: Calories 96Fat 6.1 carbohydrates 5.gSugar 2.2 protein 6.1 cholesterol 86 mg

25. **Super Easy Chocolate Chaffles**

Preparation time: 10 minutes

Cooking Time:5 minutes

Servings: 2

Ingredients:

- 1/4 cup unsweetened chocolate chips
- 1 egg
- 2 tbsps. almond flour
- 1/2 cup mozzarella cheese
- 1 tbsp. Greek yogurts
- 1/2 tsp. baking powder
- 1 tsp. stevia

Directions:

1. Switch on your square chaffle maker.
2. Spray the waffle maker with cooking spray.
3. Mix together all recipe ingredients in a mixing bowl.
4. Spoon batter in a greased waffle maker and make two chaffles.
5. Once chaffles are cooked, remove from the maker.
6. Serve with coconut cream, shredded chocolate, and nuts on top.

7. Enjoy!

Nutrition: Protein: 35% 59 kcal Fat: 59% 99 kcal Carbohydrates: 6% 10 kcal

MORE KETO CHAFFLE RECIPES

26. Maple Pumpkin Keto Chaffle Recipe

Preparation time: 10 minutes

Cooking Time: 16 Minutes

Servings: 2

Ingredients:

- 2 eggs
- 3/4 tsp baking powder
- 2 tsp pumpkin puree (100% pumpkin)
- 3/4 tsp pumpkin pie spice
- 4 tsp heavy whipping cream
- 2 tsp Lakanto Sugar-Free Maple Syrup
- 1 tsp coconut flour
- 1/2 cup mozzarella cheese, shredded
- 1/2 tsp vanilla
- Pinch of salt

Directions:

1. Turn on chaffle maker.

2. In a small bowl, combine all ingredients.

3. Cover the dash mini waffle maker with 1/4 of the batter and cook for 4 minutes.

4. Repeat 3 more times until you have made Maple Syrup Pumpkin Keto Waffles (Chaffles).

5. Serve with sugar-free maple syrup or keto ice cream.

Nutrition: (per serving):Calories: 201kcal;Carbohydrates:4g;Protein: 12g;Fat: 15g;Saturated Fat:8g;Cholesterol:200mg;Sodium:249mg;Potassium: 271mg;Fiber: 1g;Sugar: 1g;Vitamin A: 1341IU;Calcium: 254mg;Iron: 1mg

27. Garlic Bread Chaffles

Preparation time: 10 minutes

Cooking Time: 11 Minutes

Servings: 2

Ingredients:

- 1/2 cup shredded Mozzarella cheese
- 1 egg
- 1/2 tsp basil
- 1/4 tsp garlic powder
- 1 tbsp almond flour
- 1 tbsp butter
- 1/4 tsp garlic powder
- 1/4 cup shredded mozzarella cheese

Directions:

1. Heat up your Dash mini waffle maker.

2. In a small bowl, mix the egg, 1/tsp basil, 1/4 tsp garlic powder, 1 tablespoon almond flour and 1/2 cup Mozzarella Cheese.

3. Add 1/2 of the batter into your mini waffle maker and cook for 4 minutes. If they are still a bit uncooked,

leave it cooking for another 2 minutes. Then cook the rest of the batter to make a second chaffle.

4. In a small bowl, add 1 tablespoon butter and 1/tsp garlic powder and melt in the microwave. It will take about 25 seconds or so, depending on your microwave.

5. Place the chaffles on a baking sheet and use a rubber brush to spread the butter and garlic mixture on top.

6. Add 1/8th a cup of cheese on top of each chaffle.

7. Put chaffles in the oven or a toaster oven at 400 degrees and cook until the cheese is melted.

Nutrition: (per serving):Calories: 231kcal ;Carbohydrates:2g ;Protein: 13g;Fat: 19g ;Saturated Fat:10g ;Cholesterol:130mg ;Sodium:346mg ;Potassium: 52mg ;Fiber: 1g ;Sugar: 1g ;Vitamin A: 5IU ;Calcium: 232mg ;Iron: 1mg

28. Basic Keto Low Carb Chaffle Recipe

Preparation time: 10 minutes

Cooking Time: 8 Minutes

Servings: 2

Ingredients:

- 1 egg
- 1/2 cup cheddar cheese, shredded

Directions:

1. Turn waffle maker on or plug it in so that it heats and grease both sides.
2. In a small bowl, crack an egg, then add the 1/cup cheddar cheese and stir to combine.
3. Pour 1/2 of the batter in the waffle maker and close the top.
4. Cook for 3-minutes or until it reaches desired doneness.
5. Carefully remove from waffle maker and set aside for 2-3 minutes to give it time to crisp.
6. Follow the instructions again to make the second chaffle.

Nutrition: (per serving):Calories: 291kcal;Carbohydrates:1g;Protein: 20g;Fat: 23g;Saturated

Fat:13g;Cholesterol:223mg;Sodium:413mg;Potassium: 116mg;Sugar: 1g;Vitamin A: 804IU;Calcium: 432mg;Iron: 1mg

OTHER KETO CHAFFLES

29. Banana Chaffle

Preparation time: 8 minutes

Cooking Time: 16 Minutes

Servings: 2

Ingredients:

- ½ tsp banana flavoring
- 1/8 tsp salt
- 2 tbsp almond flour
- ½ shredded mozzarella cheese
- 2 eggs (beaten)
- ½ tsp baking powder
- ½ tsp cinnamon
- 2 tbsp swerve sweetener

Directions:

1. Plug the waffle maker to preheat it and spray it with a non-stick spray.

2. In a mixing bowl, combine the baking flour, cinnamon, swerve, salt, almond flour and cheese. Add the egg and

banana flavor. Mix until the ingredients are well combined.

3. Pour ¼ of the batter into your waffle maker and spread out the batter to cover all the holes on the waffle maker.

4. Close the waffle maker and cook for about minutes or according to your waffle maker's settings.

5. After the cooking cycle, use a silicone or plastic utensil to remove the chaffle from the waffle maker.

6. Repeat step 3 to 5 until you have cooked all the batter into chaffles.

7. Serve warm and enjoy.

Nutrition: Fat 12.5g 16% Carbohydrate 11g 7% Sugars 0.7g Protein 8.8g

30. __Cinnamon Roll Chaffle__

Preparation time: 10 minutes

Cooking Time: 9 Minutes

Servings: 2

Ingredients:

- 1 egg (beaten)
- ½ cup shredded mozzarella cheese
- 1 tsp cinnamon
- 1 tsp sugar free maple syrup
- ¼ tsp baking powder
- 1 tbsp almond flour
- ½ tsp vanilla extract
- Topping:
- 2 tsp granulated swerve
- 1 tbsp heavy cream
- 4 tbsp cream cheese

Directions:

1. Plug the waffle maker to preheat it and spray it with a non-stick spray.
2. In a mixing bowl, whisk together the egg, maple syrup and vanilla extract.

3. In another mixing bowl, combine the cinnamon, almond flour, baking powder and mozzarella cheese.

4. Pour in the egg mixture into the flour mixture and mix until the ingredients are well combined.

5. Pour in an appropriate amount of the batter into the waffle maker and spread out the batter to the edges to cover all the holes on the waffle maker.

6. Close the waffle maker and bake for about 3 minute or according to your waffle maker's settings.

7. After the cooking cycle, use a silicone or plastic utensil to remove the chaffle from the waffle maker.

8. Repeat step 5 to 7 until you have cooked all the batter into chaffles.

9. For the topping, combine the cream cheese, swerve and heavy cream in a microwave safe dish.

10. Place the dish in a microwave and microwave on high until the mixture is melted and smooth. Stir every 15 seconds.

11. Top the chaffles with the cream mixture and enjoy.

Nutrition: Fat 9.9g 13% Carbohydrate 3.8g 1% Sugars 0.3g Protein 4.8g

31. **Buffalo Chicken Chaffle**

Preparation time: 9 minutes

Cooking Time: 10 Minutes

Servings: 2

Ingredients:

- 1 egg
- 5 ounces cooked chicken (diced)
- 2 tbsp buffalo sauce
- ½ tsp garlic powder
- ½ tsp onion powder
- ½ tsp dried basil
- 5 tbsp shredded cheddar cheese
- 2 ounces cream cheese

Directions:

1. Plug the waffle maker and preheat it. Spray it with non-stick spray.
2. In a large mixing bowl, combine the onion powder, basil, garlic, buffalo sauce, cheddar cheese chicken and cream cheese. Mix until the ingredients are well combined and you have formed a smooth batter.

3. Sprinkle some shredded cheddar cheese over the waffle maker and pour in adequate amount of the batter. Spread out the batter to the edges of the waffle maker to cover all the holes on the waffle maker.

4. Close the lid of the waffle maker and cook for about 3 to minutes or according to waffle maker's settings.

5. After the cooking cycle, remove the chaffle from the waffle maker with a plastic or silicone utensil.

6. Repeat step 3 to 5 until you have cooked all the batter into chaffles.

7. Serve and enjoy.

Nutrition: Fat 20.1g 26% Carbohydrate 2.2g 1% Sugars 0.7g Protein 30g

32. **Pumpkin Pecan Chaffle**

Preparation time: 9 minutes

Cooking Time: 10 Minutes

Servings: 2

Ingredients:

- 2 tbsp toasted pecans (chopped)
- 2 tbsp almond flour
- 1 tbsp pumpkin puree
- ½ tsp pumpkin spice
- ½ cup grated mozzarella cheese
- 1 tsp granulated swerve sweetener
- 1 egg
- ½ tsp nutmeg
- ½ tsp vanilla extract
- ½ tsp baking powder

Directions:

1. Plug the waffle maker to preheat it and spray it with a non-stick spray.
2. In a mixing bowl, combine the almond flour, baking powder, pumpkin spice, swerve, cheese and nutmeg.

3. In another mixing bowl, whisk together the pumpkin puree egg and vanilla extract.

4. Pour the egg mixture into the flour mixture and mix until the ingredients are well combined.

5. Pour an appropriate amount of the batter into the waffle maker and spread out the batter to the edges to cover all the holes on the waffle maker.

6. Close the waffle maker and cook for about 5 minutes or according to your waffle maker's settings.

7. After the cooking cycle, use a silicone or plastic utensil to remove the chaffle from the waffle maker.

8. Repeat step 5 to 7 until you have cooked all the batter into chaffles.

9. Serve warm and top with whipped cream. Enjoy!!!

Nutrition: Fat 14.4g 18% Carbohydrate 6.3g 2% Sugars 1.4g Protein 7.5g

33. <u>Sloppy Joe Chaffle</u>

Preparation time: 9 minutes

Cooking Time: 20 Minutes

Servings: 2

Ingredients:

- Chaffle:
- 1 large egg (beaten)
- 1/8 tsp onion powder
- 1 tbsp almond flour
- ½ cup shredded mozzarella cheese
- 1 tsp nutmeg
- ¼ tsp baking powder
- Sloppy Joe Filling:
- 2 tsp olive oil
- 1 pounds ground beef
- 1 celery stalk (chopped)
- 2 tbsp ketch up
- 2 tsp Worcestershire sauce
- 1 small onions (chopped)
- 1 green bell pepper (chopped)
- 1 tbsp sugar free maple syrup

- 1 cup tomato sauce (7.9 ounce)

- 2 garlic cloves (minced)

- ½ tsp salt or to taste

- ½ tsp ground black pepper or to taste

Directions:

1. For the chaffle:

2. Plug the waffle maker and preheat it. Spray it with non-stick spray.

3. Combine the baking powder, nutmeg, flour and onion powder in a mixing bowl. Add the eggs and mix.

4. Add the cheese and mix until the ingredients are well combined and you have formed a smooth batter.

5. Pour the batter into the waffle maker and spread it out to the edges of the waffle maker to cover all the holes on it.

6. Close the waffle lid and cook for about 5 minutes or according to waffle maker's settings.

7. After the cooking cycle, remove the chaffle from the waffle maker with a plastic or silicone utensil. Transfer the chaffle to a wire rack to cool.

8. For the sloppy joe filling:

9. Heat up a large skillet over medium to high heat.

10. Add the ground beef and saute until the beef is browned.

11. Use a slotted spoon to transfer the ground beef to a paper towel lined plate to drain. Drain all the grease in the skillet.

12. Add the olive oil to the skillet and heat it up.

13. Add the onions, green pepper, celery and garlic. Sauté until the veggies are tender, stirring often to prevent burning.

14. Stir in the tomato sauce, Worcestershire sauce, ketchup, maple syrup, salt and pepper.

15. Add the browned beef and bring the mixture to a boil. Reduce the heat and simmer for about 10 minutes.

16. Remove the skillet from heat.

17. Scoop the sloppy joe into the chaffles and enjoy.

Nutrition: Fat 30.5g 39% Carbohydrate 26.2g 10% Sugars 15.3g Protein 80.2g

34. Cauliflower rice Chaffle

Preparation time: 9 minutes

Cooking Time: 8 Minutes

Ingredients:

- 1 cup cauliflower rice
- ¼ tsp salt or to taste
- 1 tbsp melted butter
- 1 egg
- ¼ tsp nutmeg
- ¼ tsp cinnamon
- ¼ tsp garlic powder
- 1/8 tsp ground black pepper or to taste
- 1/8 tsp white pepper or to taste
- ¼ tsp Italian seasoning
- ½ cup shredded parmesan cheese
- ½ cup shredded mozzarella cheese
- Garnish:
- Chopped green onions

Directions:

1. Pour ¼ of the parmesan cheese into a blender, add the mozzarella cheese, egg, salt, nutmeg, butter, cinnamon,

garlic powder, black pepper, white pepper, Italian seasoning and cauliflower.

2. Add the egg and blend until you form a smooth batter.

3. Plug the waffle maker and preheat it. Spray the waffle maker with a non-stick spray.

4. Sprinkle about tbsp of the remaining parmesan cheese on top of the waffle maker.

5. Fill the waffle maker with ¼ of the batter and spread out the batter to cover all the holes on the waffle maker. Sprinkle some shredded parmesan over the batter.

6. Close the lid of the waffle maker and cook for about 4 to 5 minutes or according to your waffle maker's settings.

7. After the cooking cycle, remove the waffle with a rubber or silicone utensil.

8. Repeat step 4 to 7 until you have cooked all the batter into chaffles.

9. Serve and enjoy.

Nutrition: Fat 15.8g 20% .Carbohydrate 6.2g 2% .Sugars 2.4g. Protein 15g

35. Chaffle And Cheese Sandwich

Preparation time: 10 minutes

Cooking Time:5 minutes

Servings: 2

Ingredients:

- 1 egg
- ½ cup mozzarella cheese
- 1 tsp. baking powder
- 3 slice feta cheese for topping

Directions:

1. Make 6 minutes chaffles
2. Set feta cheese between two chaffles.
3. Serve with hot coffee and enjoy!

Nutrition: Protein: 31% 56 kcal Fat: 60% 110 kcal Carbohydrates: 9% 16 kcal

36. Simple Chaffles With Cream Dip

Preparation time: 9 minutes

Cooking Time: 10 Minutes

Servings: 2

Ingredients:

- Chaffles
- 1 organic egg, beaten
- 2 tablespoons almond flour
- ½ teaspoon organic baking powder
- ½ cup mozzarella cheese, shredded
- Dip
- ¼ cup heavy whipping cream
- 1-2 drops liquid stevia

Directions:

1. Preheat a mini waffle iron and then grease it.
2. For chaffles: In a medium bowl, put all ingredients and with a fork, mix until well combined. Place half of the mixture into preheated waffle iron and cook for about 3–5 minutes.
3. Repeat with the remaining mixture.

4. Meanwhile, for dip: in a bowl, mix together the cream and stevia.

5. Serve warm chaffles alongside the cream dip.

Nutrition: Calories 149 Net Carbs 1.9 g Total Fat 12.8 g Saturated Fat 5.1 g Cholesterol 10mg Sodium 80 mg Total Carbs 2.7 g Fiber 0.8 g Sugar 0.4 g Protein 5.1 g

37. <u>Raspberry Chaffle</u>

Preparation time: 5 minutes

Cooking Time: 8 Minutes

Servings: 2

Ingredients:

- 1 large egg (beaten)
- 1 tsp cinnamon
- 2 tbsp cream cheese
- ½ tsp vanilla extract
- 2 tbsp heavy cream
- 2 tbsp almond flour
- ¼ tsp baking powder
- 1/3 cup raspberries
- 2 tsp swerve sweetener or to taste
- 1/8 tsp salt

Directions:

1. Plug the waffle maker to preheat it and spray it with a non-stick spray.

2. In a medium mixing bowl, combine the cinnamon, almond flour, baking powder, 1 tsp swerve and salt.

3. In another mixing bowl, combine the cream cheese, egg and vanilla extract.

4. Pour the cream cheese mixture into the cheese mixture and mix until well combine and you have formed a smooth batter.

5. Fold in half of the raspberries.

6. Fill the waffle maker with an appropriate amount of the batter. Spread out the batter to cover all the holes on the waffle maker.

7. Close the waffle maker and cook for about 3-4 minutes or according to waffle maker's settings.

8. After the cooking cycle, use a plastic or silicone utensil to remove the chaffle from the waffle maker.

9. Repeat 6 to 7 until you have cooked all the batter into chaffles.

10. In a mixing bowl, combine the remaining swerve and heavy cream. Whisk until you form soft peak.

11. Spread the cream cheese mixture over the chaffles and top with the remaining raspberries.

12. Serve and enjoy.

Nutrition: Fat 30.4g 39% Carbohydrate 16.4g 6% Sugars 3.1g Protein 12g

38. **Keto Blueberry Chaffle**

Preparation time: 5 minutes

Cooking Time: 5 Minutes

Servings: 2

Ingredients:

- ¼ cups frozen blueberries
- 1 tbsp swerve
- ½ cup shredded mozzarella cheese
- 1 tbsp almond flour
- 1 egg (beaten)
- ½ tsp ground ginger
- ½ tsp vanilla extract
- Topping:
- ½ cup heavy cream
- 1 tsp cinnamon

Directions:

1. Plug the waffle maker to preheat it and spray it with non-stick spray.
2. In a large mixing bowl, combine the swerve, almond flour and ginger. Add the egg, vanilla extract and cheese. Mix until the ingredients are well combined.

3. Gently fold in the blueberries.

4. Fill the waffle maker with the batter and spread it out to the edges of the waffle maker to cover all the holes on it.

5. Cover the lid of the waffle maker and bake for about minutes or according to waffle maker's settings.

6. After the cooking cycle, remove the chaffle from the waffle maker using a plastic or silicone utensil.

7. Repeat step 4 to 6 until you have cooked all the batter into waffles.

8. Combine the heavy whipping cream and cinnamon in a mixing bowl.

9. Top the chaffle with the heavy cream mixture and serve.

10. Enjoy.

Nutrition: Fat 29.3g 38% Carbohydrate 12.5g 5% Sugars 4.4g Protein 2g

39. Choco Peanut Butter Chaffle

Preparation time: 9 minutes

Cooking Time: 10 Minutes

Servings: 2

Ingredients:

- Filling:
- 3 tbsp all-natural peanut butter
- 2 tsp swerve sweetener
- 1 tsp vanilla extract
- 2 tbsp heavy cream
- Chaffle:
- ¼ tsp baking powder
- 1 tbsp unsweetened cocoa powder
- 4 tsp almond flour
- ½ tsp vanilla extract
- 1 tbsp granulated swerve sweetener
- 1 large egg (beaten)
- 1 tbsp heavy cream

Directions:

1. For the chaffle:

2. Plug the waffle maker and preheat it. Spray it with a non-stick spray.

3. In a large mixing bowl, combine the almond flour, cocoa powder, baking powder and swerve.

4. Add the egg, vanilla extract and heavy cream. Mix until the ingredients are well combined and you form a smooth batter.

5. Pour some of the batter into the preheated waffle maker. Spread out the batter to the edges of the waffle maker to cover all the holes on the waffle iron.

6. Close the lid of the waffle iron and bake for about 5 minutes or according to waffle maker's settings.

7. After the baking cycle, use a plastic or silicone utensil to remove the chaffle from the waffle maker.

8. Repeat step 4 to 6 until you have cooked all the batter into chaffles.

9. Transfer the chaffles to a wire rack and let the chaffles cool completely.

10. For the filling:

11. Combine the vanilla, swerve, heavy cream and peanut butter in a bowl. Mix until the ingredients are well combined.

12. Spread the peanut butter frosting over the chaffles and serve.

13. Enjoy.

Nutrition: Fat 43.2g 55% Carbohydrate 32g12% Sugars 9g Protein 19g

40. <u>Avocado Chaffles</u>

Servings:2

Cooking Time: 5 Minutes

Ingredients:

- 1 large egg
- 1/2 cup finely shredded mozzarella
- 1/8 cup avocado mash
- 1 tbsp. coconut cream
- TOPPING
- 2 oz. smoked salmon
- 1 Avocado thinly sliced

Directions:

1. Switch on your square waffle maker and grease with cooking spray.
2. Beat egg in a mixing bowl with a fork.
3. Add the cheese, avocado mash and coconut cream to the egg and mix well.
4. Pour chaffle mixture in the preheated waffle maker and cook for about 2-3 minutes Utes.
5. Once chaffles are cooked, carefully remove from the maker.

6. Serve with an avocado slice and smoked salmon.

7. Drizzle ground pepper on top.

8. Enjoy!

Nutrition: Protein: 23% kcal Fat: 67% 266 kcal Carbohydrates: 11% 42 kcal

41. <u>Almond Butter Chaffle</u>

Preparation time: 8 minutes

Cooking Time: 20 Minutes

Servings: 2

Ingredients:

- 2 eggs (beaten)
- 3 tsp granulated swerve sweetener
- 4 tbsp almond flour
- ½ tsp vanilla extract
- ½ cup grated mozzarella cheese
- ½ cup parmesan cheese
- 1/8 tsp allspice
- Almond Butter Filling:
- ½ tsp vanilla extract
- 4 tbsp almond butter
- 2 tbsp butter (melted)
- 2 tbsp swerve sweetener
- 1/8 tsp nutmeg

Directions:

1. Plug the waffle maker to preheat it and spray it with a non-stick cooking spray.

2. In a mixing bowl, combine the mozzarella, allspice, almond flour, and swerve sweetener. Add the egg and vanilla extract and mix until the ingredients are well combined.

3. Sprinkle some parmesan cheese over the waffle maker.

4. Pour an appropriate amount of the batter into the waffle and spread out the batter to cover all the holes on the waffle maker.

5. Sprinkle some parmesan over the batter.

6. Close the waffle maker and cook for about 5 minutes or according to your waffle maker's settings.

7. After the cooking cycle, use a plastic or silicone utensil to remove the chaffle from the waffle maker. Transfer the chaffle to a wire rack to cool.

8. Repeat step 3 to 7 until you have cooked all the batter into chaffles.

9. For the filling, combine butter, almond butter, swerve, vanilla and nutmeg. Mix until the mixture is smooth and fluffy.

10. Spread the cream over the surface of one chaffle and cover the with another chaffle. Repeat until you have filled all the chaffles.

11. Serve and enjoy.

Nutrition: Fat 54.8g 70% Carbohydrate 18.4g7% Sugars 3.2g Protein 29.7g

42. Simple Chaffles Without Maker

Servings:2

Cooking Time:5minutes

Ingredients:

- 1 tbsp. chia seeds
- 1 egg
- 1/2 cup cheddar cheese
- pinch of salt
- 1 tbsp. avocado oil

Directions:

1. Heat your nonstick pan over medium heat
2. In a small bowl, mix together chia seeds, salt, egg, and cheese together
3. Grease pan with avocado oil.
4. Once the pan is hot, pour 2 tbsps. chaffle batter and cook for about 1-2 minutes Utes.
5. Flip and cook for another 1-2 minutes Utes.
6. Once chaffle is brown remove from pan.
7. Serve with berries on top and enjoy.

Nutrition: Protein: 19% 44 kcal Fat: % 181 kcal Carbohydrates: 1% 2 kcal

43. Heart Shape Chaffles

Servings:2

Cooking Time:5 Minutes

Ingredients:

- 1 egg
- 1 cup mozzarella cheese
- 1 tsp baking powder
- ¼ cup almond flour
- 1 tbsp. coconut oil

Directions:

1. Heat your nonstick pan over medium heat.
2. Mix together all ingredients in a bowl.
3. Grease pan with avocado oil and place a heart shape cookie cutter over the pan.
4. Once the pan is hot, pour the batter equally in 2 cutters.
5. Cook for another 1-2 minutes Utes.
6. Once chaffle is set, remove the cutter, flip and cook for another 1-2 minutes Utes.
7. Once chaffles are brown, remove from the pan.
8. Serve hot and enjoy!

Nutrition: Protein: 24% 43 kcal Fat: 6 123 kcal Carbohydrates: 6% 11 kcal

44. **Bacon Chaffles With Herb Dip**

Preparation time: 9 minutes

Cooking Time: 10 Minutes

Servings: 2

Ingredients:

- Chaffles
- 1 organic egg, beaten
- ½ cup Swiss/Gruyere cheese blend, shredded
- 2 tablespoons cooked bacon pieces
- 1 tablespoon jalapeño pepper, chopped
- Dip
- ¼ cup heavy cream
- ¼ teaspoon fresh dill, minced
- Pinch of ground black pepper

Directions:

1. Preheat a mini waffle iron and then grease it.
2. For chaffles: In a medium bowl, put all ingredients and mix well.
3. Place half of the mixture into preheated waffle iron and cook for about 5 minutes.
4. Repeat with the remaining mixture.

5. Meanwhile, for dip: in a bowl, mix together the cream and stevia.

6. Serve warm chaffles alongside the dip.

Nutrition: Calories 210   Net Carbs 2.2 g Total Fat 13 g Saturated Fat 9.7 g   Cholesterol 132 mg   Sodium 164 mg Total Carbs 2.3 g Fiber 0.1 g Sugar 0.7 g Protein 11.9 g

45. Broccoli Chaffles On Pan

Servings:4

Cooking Time:5 Minutes

Ingredients:

- 1 egg
- 1 cup cheddar cheese
- ½ cup broccoli chopped
- 1 tsp baking powder
- 1 pinch garlic powder
- 1 pinch salt
- 1 pinch black pepper
- 1 tbsp. coconut oil

Directions:

1. Heat your nonstick pan over medium heat.
2. Mix together all ingredients in a bowl.
3. Grease pan with oil.
4. Once the pan is hot, pour broccoli and cheese batter on greased pan
5. Cook for 1-2 minutes Utes.
6. Flip and cook for another 1-2 minutes Utes.
7. Once chaffles are brown, remove from the pan.

8. Serve with raspberries and melted coconut oil on top.

9. Enjoy!

Nutrition: Protein: 20% 40 kcal Fat: 72% 142 kcal Carbohydrates: 7% 15 kcal

46. Chicken Chaffles With Tzatziki

Preparation time: 9 minutes

Cooking Time: 12 Minutes

Servings: 2

Ingredients:

- Chaffles
- 1 organic egg, beaten
- 1/3 cup grass-fed cooked chicken, chopped
- 1/3 cup mozzarella cheese, shredded
- ¼ teaspoon garlic, minced
- ¼ teaspoon dried basil, crushed
- Tzatziki
- ¼ cup plain Greek yogurt
- ½ of small cucumber, peeled, seeded, and chopped
- 1 teaspoon olive oil
- ½ teaspoon fresh lemon juice
- Pinch of ground black pepper
- ¼ tablespoon fresh dill, chopped
- ½ of garlic clove, peeled

Directions:

1. Preheat a mini waffle iron and then grease it.

2. For chaffles: In a medium bowl, put all ingredients and with your hands, mix until well combined. Place half of the mixture into preheated waffle iron and cook for about 4–6 minutes.
3. Repeat with the remaining mixture.
4. Meanwhile, for tzatziki: in a food processor, place all the ingredients and pulse until well combined.
5. Serve warm chaffles alongside the tzatziki.

Nutrition: Calories 131 Net Carbs 4.4 g Total Fat 5 g Saturated Fat 2 g Cholesterol 104 mg Sodium 97 mg Total Carbs 4.7 g Fiber 0.3 g Sugar 3 g Protein 13 g

47. Cereal and Walnut Chaffle

Preparation time: 9 minutes

Cooking Time: 6 Minutes

Ingredients:

- 1 milliliter of cereal flavoring
- ¼ tsp baking powder
- 1 tsp granulated swerve
- 1/8 tsp xanthan gum
- 1 tbsp butter (melted)
- ½ tsp coconut flour
- 2 tbsp toasted walnut (chopped)
- 1 tbsp cream cheese
- 2 tbsp almond flour
- 1 large egg (beaten)
- ¼ tsp cinnamon
- 1/8 tsp nutmeg

Directions:

1. Plug the waffle maker to preheat it and spray it with a non-stick spray.
2. In a mixing bowl, whisk together the egg, cereal flavoring, cream cheese and butter.

3. In another mixing bowl, combine the coconut flour, almond flour, cinnamon, nutmeg, swerve, xanthan gum and baking powder.

4. Pour the egg mixture into the flour mixture and mix until you form a smooth batter.

5. Fold in the chopped walnuts.

6. Pour in an appropriate amount of the batter into the waffle maker and spread out the batter to the edges to cover all the holes on the waffle maker.

7. Close the waffle maker and cook for about 3 minutes or according to your waffle maker's settings.

8. After the cooking cycle, use a plastic or silicone utensil to remove the chaffle from the waffle maker.

9. Repeat step 6 to 8 until you have cooked all the batter into chaffles.

10. Serve and top with sour cream or heavy cream.

Nutrition: Fat 18.2g 23% Carbohydrate 4.7g 2% Sugars 0.6g Protein 7.1g

48. Chaffle With Cream and Salmon

Preparation time: 8 minutes

Cooking Time: 20 Minutes

Servings: 2

Ingredients:

- 1/2 medium onion sliced
- 2 tbsps. parsley chopped
- 4 oz. smoked salmon
- 4 tbsp. heavy cream
- CHAFFLE Ingredients:
- 1 egg
- 1/2 cup mozzarella cheese
- 1 tsp stevia
- 1 tsp vanilla
- 2 tbsps. almond flour

Directions:

1. Make 4 Heart shape chaffles with the chaffle ingredients
2. Arrange smoked salmon and heavy cream on each Chaffle.
3. Top with onion slice and parsley.

4. Serve as it is and enjoy!

Nutrition: Protein: 34% 79 kcal Fat: 60% 137 kcal Carbohydrates: 6% 14 kcal

Fat: 70% 133 kcal Carbohydrates: 5% 9 kcal

49. Cornbread Chaffle

Preparation time: 10 minutes

Cooking Time: 12 Minutes

Servings: 2

Ingredients:

- 1 ½ tbsp melted butter
- 3 tbsp almond flour
- 1 milliliter cornbread flavoring
- 2 tbsp Mexican blend cheese
- 2 tbsp shredded parmesan cheese
- 1 small jalapeno (seeded and sliced)
- 2 tsp swerve sweetener
- 1 large egg (beaten)
- ½ tsp all spice

Directions:

1. Plug the waffle maker to preheat it and spray it with a non-stick cooking spray.
2. In a mixing bowl, combine almond flour, jalapeno, all spice, baking powder and swerve.
3. In another mixing bowl, whisk together the egg, butter and cornbread flavoring.

4. Pour the egg mixture into the flour mixture and mix until you form a smooth batter. Stir in the cheese.

5. Sprinkle some parmesan cheese over the waffle maker. Pour an appropriate amount of the batter into the waffle maker and spread out the batter to the edges to cover all the holes on the waffle maker. Sprinkle some parmesan over the batter

6. Close the waffle maker and bake for about 5 minutes or according to you waffle maker's settings.

7. After the baking cycle, remove the chaffle from the waffle maker with a plastic or silicone utensil.

8. Repeat step 5 to 7 until you have cooked all the batter into chaffles.

9. Serve warm with your desired topping and enjoy.

Nutrition: Fat 13.6g 17% Carbohydrate 4.1g 1% Sugars 0.8g Protein 6.4g

50. <u>Midday Chaffle Snacks</u>

Preparation time: 8 minutes

Cooking Time: 5 Minutes

Ingredients:

- 4 minutes Chaffles
- 2 oz. coconut flakes
- 2 oz. kiwi slice
- 2 oz. raspberry
- 2 oz. almonds chopped
- CHAFFLE Ingredients:
- 1 egg
- 1/2 cup mozzarella cheese
- 1 tsp stevia
- 1 tsp vanilla
- 2 tbsps. almond flour

Directions:

1. Make 4 minutes chaffles with the chaffle ingredients.
2. Arrange coconut flakes, raspberries, almonds and raspberries on each chaffle.
3. Serve and enjoy keto snacks

Nutrition: Protein: 18% 37 kcal Fat: 67% 137 kcal Carbohydrates: 15% 31 kc

CONCLUSION

The most documented benefit of a keto diet is rapid weight loss. Contrary to belief, many people have described becoming less hungry. Also, keto can minimize acne, and it can even increase heart protection and maintain neural activity, either way, you may want to contact a doctor to get his opinion and guidelines once you start buying avocado boxes and especially if you have problems with obesity. Everyone's requirements are different and it doesn't fit you individually what works for the vast majority of citizens. When choosing foods, you can not only look at the fat quality but also evaluate the protein. In your keto diet, you only need protein moderately - about 20 percent of your total calorie consumption can come from protein - and some nuts seem to be rich in protein.

From a mineral and vitamin perspective, make sure to incorporate fiber-rich fruits and vegetables like cabbage, broccoli, and cauliflower.

The transition into ketosis takes about 2-4 days depending on the person (assuming carbs are low enough). The amount of carbohydrate needed to reach ketosis can also vary from person to person. "The initial weight loss will be very rapid, but keep in mind that much of it will be in glycogen (carbs) and water. This is followed by a slow weight loss due to the lack of calories and the consumption of more fat than fuel." As the saying goes, slow and steady wins the race, and this is extremely valid for diets. You'll lose weight easily on keto, but you may need to pay attention to the long-term results so your body can adapt to your new diet.

Without a doubt, chaffs have dominated the world of low carb dieting: they're awesome. For unlimited combinations of condiments, sweet or savory, you can add and change a very simple ingredient with just cheese and eggs. Use them individually or as a source of seasonings and toppings. A simple calculation of chaffle is 1/2 cup with 1 egg of cheese for each chaffle. Start adding coconut flour or almond flour. Experiment around with the cheeses. Add veggies, berries, spices or nuts and let your imagination run wild.

Chaffles can be frozen and processed, so a large quantity can be made and stored for quick and extremely fast meals. If you don't have a waffle iron, simply bake the mixture like a pancake in a skillet, or even cooler, in a deep fryer. You won't get the fluffy sides like you do with a waffle iron, but they will definitely taste great. Depending on which cheese you choose, the carbs and net calorie count may shift a bit. In general, though, the waffles are completely carb-free, whether you use real whole milk cheese or not. Waffles will keep frozen for up to a month. However, they absorb a lot of moisture when thawed, making it difficult to get them crispy again. Chaffles are high in fat, moderate in protein and low in carbohydrates. Chaffles are a very proven and popular technique for keeping people on board. And chaffles are more shelf-stable and better than most forms of keto bread. "Whatever high-carb diet you might want. A non-stick waffle iron is something that makes life easier, and it's a trade-off we're happy to make for our well-being.

In summary, the keto diet is healthy and helpful for your well being and weight reduction if you are very conscientious and conscious about it. The best way to monitor your keto commitment is to use a diet tracking app where you simply set the target amount of macronutrients / macro breakdown (on keto it would definitely be 75 percent fat, 5 percent carbs and 20 percent protein) and check the labels of the foods you consume.

With everything, as with any lifestyle change, allow yourself some time to acclimate. You'll see some quick changes almost immediately, but to keep the weight off, you need to stick with the plan, even if the improvement slows down a bit. Slowing down doesn't mean the new diet is no longer working; it just means your body is adjusting to the new diet. Weight loss, or something like losing the unnecessary excess weight, is just a side result of a healthy, better lifestyle that can support you in the long run, not just the short run.

CPSIA information can be obtained
at www.ICGtesting.com
Printed in the USA
LVHW020414120521
687183LV00009B/848

9 781802 858549